PANCREATITIS DIET

COOKBOOK

Delicious And Easy Recipes to Prevent

and Reserve Pancreatitis

Copyright © 2021

DISCLAIMER

Please note that the information and recipes in this book are written for the express purpose of sharing educational information only. The information herein is stated to be reliable and consistence, but the author neither implies nor intends any guarantee of accuracy for specific cases or individuals.

It is recommended that you consult a licensed professional before beginning any practise relating to your diet or lifestyle. The contents of this book are not replacement for professional advice.

The author, publisher and distributors disclaim any liability, loss or damage and risk taken by individuals who directly or indirectly act on the information contained in this book.

Table of Contents

Introduction

Pancreatitis is a condition characterized by inflammation of the pancreas. The pancreas is a large organ behind the stomach that produces digestive enzymes and a number of hormones. Because the pancreas is so closely tied to your digestive process, it's affected by what you choose to eat. In cases of acute pancreatitis, pancreas inflammation is often triggered by gallstones. But in cases of chronic pancreatitis in which flare ups recur overtime, your diet might have a lot to do with the problem.

Not only is following a diet for pancreatitis neccessary to help recover, but it is very important to help prevent this disease from entering chronic phase.

To get your pancreas healthy, focus on foods that are rich in protein, low in animal fats, and contain antioxidants. Try lean meats, beans and lentils, clear soups, and dairy alternatives (such as flax milk and almond milk). Your pancreas won't have to work as hard to process these.

Research suggests that some people with pancreatitis can tolerate up to 30 to 40% of calories from fat when it's from whole-food plant sources or medium-chain triglycerides (MCTs). Others do better with much lower fat intake, such as 50 grams or less per day.

Spinach, blueberries, cherries, and whole grains can work to protect your digestion and fight the free radicals that damage your organs.

If you're craving something sweet, reach for fruit instead of added sugars since those with pancreatitis are at high risk for diabetes.

Consider cherry tomatoes, cucumbers and hummus, and fruit as your go-to snacks. Your pancreas will thank you.

Foods to limit include:

- red meat
- organ meats
- fried foods
- fries and potato chips
- mayonnaise
- margarine and butter
- full-fat dairy
- pastries and desserts with added sugars
- beverages with added sugars

If you're trying to combat pancreatitis, avoid trans-fatty acids in your diet.

Fried or heavily processed foods, like french fries and fast-food hamburgers, are some of the

worst offenders. Organ meats, full-fat dairy,
potato chips, and mayonnaise also top the list of
foods to limit.

 Cooked or deep-fried foods might trigger a
flare-up of pancreatitis. You'll also want to cut
back on the refined flour found in cakes,
pastries, and cookies. These foods can tax the
digestive system by causing your insulin levels
to spike.

Pancreatitis recovery diet

If you're recovering from acute or chronic
pancreatitis, avoid drinking alcohol. If you
smoke, you'll also need to quit. Focus on eating
a low-fat diet that won't tax or inflame your
pancreas.

 You should also stay hydrated. Keep an
electrolyte beverage or a bottle of water with
you at all times.

If you've been hospitalized due to a pancreatitis flare-up, your doctor will probably refer you to a dietitian to help you learn how to change your eating habits permanently.

People with chronic pancreatitis often experience malnutrition due to their decreased pancreas function. Vitamins A, D, E, and K are most commonly found to be lacking as a result of pancreatitis.

Diet tips

Always check with your doctor or dietician before changing your eating habits when you have pancreatitis. Here are some tips they might suggest:

Eat between six and eight small meals throughout the day to help recover from pancreatitis. This is easier on your digestive system than eating two or three large meals.

Use MCTs as your primary fat since this type of fat does not require pancreatic enzymes to be digested. MCTs can be found in coconut oil and palm kernel oil and is available at most health food stores.

Avoid eating too much fiber at once, as this can slow digestion and result in less-than-ideal absorption of nutrients from food. Fiber may also make your limited amount of enzymes less effective.

Take a multivitamin supplement to ensure that you're getting the nutrition you need. You can find a great selection of multivitamins here.

Causes of pancreatitis

The most common cause of chronic pancreatitis is drinking too much alcohol, according to the U.S. Department of Health and Human Services.

Pancreatitis can also be genetic, or the symptom of an autoimmune reaction. In many cases of acute pancreatitis, the condition is triggered by a blocked bile duct or gallstones.

Other treatments for pancreatitis

If your pancreas has been damaged by pancreatitis, a change in your diet will help you feel better. But it might not be enough to restore the function of the pancreas completely.

Your doctor may prescribe supplemental or synthetic pancreatic enzymes for you to take with every meal.

If you're still experiencing pain from chronic pancreatitis, consider alternative therapy such as yoga or acupuncture to supplement your doctor's prescribed pancreatitis treatment.

Recipes

Prep:8 mins

Cook:10 mins - 12 mins

Easy

Makes 6

Bake our easy bread thins with wholemeal spelt and top with your favourite ingredients. We have ideas for using them in two healthy lunch recipes

Ingredients

- 190g plain wholemeal spelt flour , plus extra for dusting
- ½ tsp bicarbonate of soda
- 1 tsp baking powder
- 75ml live bio yogurt made up to 150ml with cold water

Method

1. Heat oven to 200C/180C fan/gas 6 and line a baking sheet with baking parchment. Mix the flour, bicarbonate of soda and baking powder in a bowl, then stir in the diluted yogurt with the blade of a knife until you have a soft, sticky dough, adding a little water if the mix is dry.

2. Tip the dough onto a lightly floured surface and shape and flatten with your hands to make a 20cm round. Take care not to over-handle as it can make the bread tough. Lift onto the baking sheet and cut into six triangles, slightly easing them apart with the knife. Bake for about 10-12 mins – they don't have to be golden, but should feel firm. Leave to cool on a wire rack.

3. Use to make our wild salmon & avocado triangles and goat's cheese, tomato & olive triangles. The rest can be packed

into a food bag to use later in the week, or frozen until needed.

Sausage ragu

Prep:5 mins

Cook:45 mins

Easy

Serves 4

Feed the family this comforting, budget-friendly sausage ragu with pasta. You can freeze the leftovers for another time and it tastes just as good

Ingredients

- 3 tbsp olive oil
- 1 onion, finely chopped
- 2 large garlic cloves, crushed
- ¼ tsp chilli flakes
- 2 rosemary sprigs, leaves finely chopped
- 2 x 400g cans chopped tomatoes

- 1 tbsp brown sugar

- 6 pork sausages

- 150ml whole milk

- 1 lemon, zested

- 350g rigatoni pasta

- grated parmesan and ½ small bunch parsley, leaves roughly chopped, to serve

Method

1. Heat 2 tbsp of the oil in a saucepan over a medium heat. Fry the onion with a pinch of salt for 7 mins. Add the garlic, chilli and rosemary, and cook for 1 min more. Tip in the tomatoes and sugar, and simmer for 20 mins.

2. Heat the remaining oil in a medium frying pan over a medium heat. Squeeze the sausagemeat from the skins and fry, breaking it up with a wooden spoon, for 5-7 mins until golden. Add to the sauce with the milk and lemon zest, then

simmer for a further 5 mins. To freeze,
leave to cool completely and transfer to
large freezerproof bags.

3. Cook the pasta following pack
   instructions. Drain and toss with the
   sauce. Scatter over the parmesan and
   parsley leaves to serve.

Prep:15 mins

Cook:20 mins

Easy

Serves 4

Cook up this classic sauce in one pan, then toss
with spaghetti for a simple midweek meal. It's
budget-friendly too, making it a great meal for
the family

Ingredients

- 3 tbsp olive oil

- 1 onion, finely chopped

- 2 large garlic cloves, crushed

- ½ tsp chilli flakes (optional)

- 400g can chopped tomatoes

- 5 anchovy fillets, finely chopped

- 120g pitted black olives

- 2 tbsp capers, drained

- 300g dried spaghetti

- ½ small bunch of parsley, finely chopped

Method

1. Heat the oil in a non-stick pan over a medium-low heat. Add the onion along with a generous pinch of salt and fry for 10 mins, or until soft. Add the garlic and chilli, if using, and cook for a further minute.

2. Stir the tomatoes, anchovies, olives and capers into the onion, bring to a gentle simmer and cook, uncovered, for 15 mins. Season to taste.

3. Meanwhile, bring a large pan of salted
   water to the boil. Cook the spaghetti
   following pack instructions, then drain
   and toss with the sauce and parsley.

Chicken parmigiana

Prep:40 mins

Cook:30 mins

More effort

Serves 4

Make midweek easier with our family-friendly
chicken parmagiana. Ideal for freezing for busy
week nights, the recipe is also easily doubled

Ingredients

- large chicken breasts
- 50g plain flour
- 1 egg, beaten
- 75g fresh breadcrumbs

- 15g parmesan, finely grated, plus extra to serve
- tbsp sunflower oil
- 125g ball mozzarella, cut into 4 slices
- 300g spaghetti
- For the tomato sauce
- tbsp olive oil
- garlic cloves, finely sliced
- pinch of caster sugar
- splash of red wine vinegar
- x 400g cans chopped tomatoes or passata
- 1 tsp dried oregano

Method

1. Cut each chicken breast in half lengthways so you have four fillets. Put the fillets on a board, cover with a sheet of baking parchment and bash with a rolling pin until they are the same thickness all over.

2. Put the flour in a shallow dish and season with a little salt. Tip the egg into another dish, then the breadcrumbs and parmesan into a third dish, stirring to combine. Working with one chicken fillet at a time, coat in the flour, then dip into the beaten egg, and finally coat in the cheesy breadcrumb mixture. Transfer the breadcrumbed fillets to a plate as you go. To freeze, stack the fillets in a freezerproof container between sheets of baking parchment. Will keep frozen for three months.

3. To make the sauce, heat the olive oil in a shallow pan and sizzle the garlic for 2 mins. Sprinkle in the sugar and add a splash of the vinegar, then tip in the tomatoes or passata. Add the oregano, season and bubble for 10-15 mins, stirring occasionally until thickened. To freeze, leave to cool completely, then transfer to

a freezerproof container (portion it into
more than one, if you like). Will keep
frozen for up to three months. Defrost
overnight in the fridge, then reheat in a
pan until piping hot.

4. Heat the sunflower oil in a large frying
pan over a medium heat and cook the
breadcrumbed chicken fillets for 3 mins
on each side (fresh or from frozen) until
golden and crisp. Arrange on a baking
tray. Spoon a little of the sauce over the
middle of each fillet, and top each with a
slice of mozzarella. Heat the grill to high.
Cook the spaghetti following pack
instructions, then drain and toss with the
remaining sauce. Grill the fillets for 3-4
mins, or 1-2 mins more if they're from the
freezer, until the mozzarella is melted and
bubbling, then serve.

Prep:10 mins

Cook:2 hrs and 10 mins

Easy

Serves 4 with leftovers

Pot-roast your chicken to ensure that it's succulent. This recipe will also give you an amazing stock to use in other recipes so it's a winner all round

Ingredients

- 2 tbsp olive oil
- 2.4kg chicken – buy the best you can afford
- 4 onions, peeled and cut into large wedges
- ½ bunch thyme
- 3 garlic cloves
- 6 peppercorns
- 175ml white wine

* 1.2l chicken stock

Method

1. Heat oven to 170C/150C fan/gas 5. Heat
   the oil in a large flameproof casserole dish
   and brown the chicken well on all sides,
   then sit it breast-side up. Pack in the
   onions, thyme, garlic and peppercorns,
   pour over the wine and stock, and bring
   to the boil. Pop on the lid and transfer to
   the oven for 2 hrs.

2. Remove and rest for 20 mins. Carefully
   lift the chicken onto a chopping board
   and carve as much as you need. Serve the
   carved chicken in a shallow bowl with the
   onions and some of the stock poured
   over. Serve with some usual Sunday veg
   and roast potatoes.

3. Strain the leftover stock into a bowl and
   strip the carcass of all the chicken. Chill
   both for up to three days or freeze for up

to a month to use for other recipes like our one-pot chicken noodle soup.

RECIPE TIPS

USE THE LEFTOVERS

1. Use the stock and chicken from this recipe to make chicken & leek filo pie, one-pot Chinese chicken noodle soup, or Mexican chicken & black bean wraps.

Easy sausage & fennel risotto

Prep:15 mins

Cook:45 mins

Easy

Serves 4

Warm up on chilly nights with this comforting risotto. It's a budget-friendly choice for feeding the family on busy weeknights

Ingredients

- tbsp olive oil

- 1 onion , finely chopped

- 1 fennel bulb , finely sliced

- pork sausages

- ½ tsp fennel seeds , crushed

- large garlic cloves , crushed

- thyme sprigs, leaves finely chopped, plus extra to serve

- 400g risotto rice

- 100ml white wine

- litres hot chicken stock

- 70g parmesan , finely grated

- 1 lemon , zested and juiced

Method

1. Heat the oil in a large saucepan, add the onion and fennel and fry for 10 mins or until softened. Raise the heat. Squeeze the sausagemeat out of the skins straight into the pan and fry for 5 mins, or until turning golden brown. Stir through the

fennel seeds, garlic and thyme and fry for
a further minute.

2. Tip in the rice and fry for 1 min. Pour the
   wine into the pan and boil the liquid until
   reduced by half. Add half the stock and
   cook until absorbed, stirring constantly.
   Add the remaining stock, a ladleful at a
   time, and cook until al dente and not too
   thick in consistency, stirring constantly
   for 20-25 mins. Season with black pepper.

3. Stir through the cheese and lemon, then
   spoon into four bowls and scatter over
   the extra thyme leaves to finish.

Honey & soy chicken with sesame broccoli

Prep:10 mins

Cook:45 mins

Easy

Serves 4

Enjoy these sticky honey and soy chicken thighs as part of an easy midweek meal. This budget-friendly dinner is sure to be a family favourite

Ingredients

- tbsp soy sauce
- tbsp honey
- tbsp oil
- 1 tbsp garlic & ginger paste
- 8 skin-on chicken thighs
- 1 large head broccoli , cut into florets
- 1 tbsp sesame seeds
- rice , to serve (optional)

Method

1. Heat oven to 200C/180C fan/gas 6. Mix the soy, honey, 1 tbsp of the oil and ½ tbsp garlic & ginger paste in a bowl. Pour over the chicken thighs and leave to marinate if you have time, but don't worry if not – they will be delicious either

way. Tip the chicken with all the
marinade into a roasting tin, skin-side up.
Cook for 45 mins until sticky and the skin
is crispy.

2. When the chicken has 15 mins left, start
   cooking the rice following pack
   instructions, if using, and heat the
   remaining oil in a frying pan. Add the
   remaining garlic & ginger paste, sizzle for
   1 min, then tip in the broccoli along with
   a splash of water. Cover and cook for 10
   mins until tender, then take the lid off, tip
   the sesame seeds into the pan and give
   everything a good toss around. Season.
   Serve with the chicken, and all the
   caramelised bits from the bottom of the
   tin.

Easy chocolate fudge cake

Prep:25 mins

Cook:30 mins

Easy

Serves 8

Need a guaranteed crowd-pleasing cake that's easy to make? This super-squidgy chocolate fudge cake with smooth icing is an instant baking win

Ingredients

- 150ml sunflower oil, plus extra for the tin
- 175g self-raising flour
- 2 tbsp cocoa powder
- 1 tsp bicarbonate of soda
- 150g caster sugar
- 2 tbsp golden syrup
- 2 large eggs, lightly beaten
- 150ml semi-skimmed milk
- For the icing
- 100g unsalted butter
- 225g icing sugar
- 40g cocoa powder

- 2½ tbsp milk (a little more if needed)

Method

1. Heat the oven to 180C/160C fan/gas 4. Oil and line the base of two 18cm sandwich tins. Sieve the flour, cocoa powder and bicarbonate of soda into a bowl. Add the caster sugar and mix well.

2. Make a well in the centre and add the golden syrup, eggs, sunflower oil and milk. Beat well with an electric whisk until smooth.

3. Pour the mixture into the two tins and bake for 25-30 mins until risen and firm to the touch. Remove from oven, leave to cool for 10 mins before turning out onto a cooling rack.

4. To make the icing, beat the unsalted butter in a bowl until soft. Gradually sieve and beat in the icing sugar and cocoa powder, then add enough of the milk to make the icing fluffy and spreadable.

5. Sandwich the two cakes together with the butter icing and cover the sides and the top of the cake with more icing.

Prep:5 mins

Cook:20 mins

Easy

Serves 2

A grilled omelette with sweet onion base, dotted with creamy cheese and served with salad - this recipes make enough for lunch the next day

Ingredients

- 4 tsp rapeseed oil

- 2 large red onions , finely sliced

- 4 tsp clear honey

- 8 large eggs

- 140g goat's cheese

- 100g salad leaf (such as rocket, baby leaves, watercress and spinach)

- 250g cooked beetroot , sliced

- juice ½' lemon

Method

1. Heat the grill to high. Put the oil and onions in a medium-to-large ovenproof non-stick frying pan and sweat on a low-medium heat with the lid on for about 10 mins, or until they begin to soften and brown a little at the edges. Reduce heat to low, add the honey, stir well, then leave to bubble for 1 min or so. Meanwhile, crack the eggs into a bowl and beat with a fork, then add some black pepper.

2. Pour the eggs into the pan and cook for 5-6 mins until almost set. Break the goat's cheese into large chunks and dot over the top. Place the frittata under the hot grill for 3 mins, then shake to check that the egg is set firm and the cheese is soft and bubbling. Pop it back under the grill for 1 min or so more if needed.

3. Mix the salad leaves and beetroot in a large bowl. Dress with the lemon juice and toss. Cut the frittata into quarters – cool then chill half for Frittata and salad (see 'goes well with'). Serve the rest warm with the salad on the side.

Chocolate & raspberry birthday layer cake

Prep:20 mins

Cook:40 mins

plus cooling

Easy

Serves 12

Who could resist our chocolate and raspberry cake? Like a Victoria sponge but better, try budget-friendly frozen raspberries for the cream

Ingredients

- 225ml sunflower oil , plus extra for the tins
- 250g caster sugar
- large eggs
- 225ml milk
- 250g self-raising flour
- tbsp cocoa
- 1½ tsp bicarbonate of soda
- For the raspberry layer
- 150g raspberry jam
- 100g frozen raspberries , defrosted
- 300ml double cream
- tbsp icing sugar

Method

1. Heat the oven to 180C/160C fan/gas 4. Oil and line two round 20cm springform cake tins with baking parchment. Whisk the oil, sugar, eggs and milk in a bowl until smooth. Sieve the flour, cocoa and bicarb into another large bowl, then gradually mix in the wet ingredients.

2. Divide the mixture between the tins and bake for 35-40 mins until the cakes are risen and spring back when pressed. Leave to cool in the tins for 10 mins, then transfer to a wire rack to cool completely.

3. For the raspberry layer, stir the jam and the defrosted raspberries together. Once the cakes are cool, whip the cream with the sugar to soft peaks, then gently fold half the raspberry mixture through the cream to create a ripple effect.

4. Spoon most of the reserved raspberry mixture over one of the cakes, then dollop on half of the cream. Smooth over with a

palette knife, then place the other sponge on top. Swirl over the remaining cream and swirl the last of the raspberry mixture through it. Will keep in the fridge for two days.

RECIPE TIPS

SIMPLE SWAPS

1. Making chocolate cakes and buttercream icing can be expensive, but using vegetable oil instead of butter, and cocoa instead of melted chocolate, keeps costs down. It means the cake also keeps well (it won't go stale if it's wrapped and left for a few days, or you can freeze the sponges to decorate later) and it creates a texture that ensures the layers will stack and slice beautifully. Adding lashings of whipped cream looks lavish, but it's usually more cost-effective than making buttercream.

Prep:5 mins

Cook:30 mins

Easy

Serves 4

Give student staple tuna pasta a boost with capers, mascarpone, lemon zest and parmesan for a more sophisticated take on a budget-friendly midweek meal

Ingredients

- tbsp olive oil
- 1 red onion , finely chopped
- 500g cherry tomatoes , halved
- 400g dried pasta (we used rigatoni)
- 1l hot vegetable stock
- x 110g cans tuna in olive oil, drained
- tbsp mascarpone
- 30g parmesan , grated
- heaped tbsp capers

- ½ lemon , zested

- small bunch parsley , finely chopped

Method

1. Heat the oil in a saucepan over a medium-low heat. Add the onion and a pinch of salt and fry gently for 7 mins or until softened and turning translucent. Add 350g of the tomatoes, the pasta and veg stock to the pan and bring to the boil, then reduce to a simmer and cook for 15 mins, uncovered, stirring occasionally. The tomatoes should have broken down and the pasta will be just cooked.

2. Add the remaining tomatoes and bubble uncovered on a medium-high heat for 5 mins or until the liquid has reduced. Gently fold through large flakes of tuna, the mascarpone, parmesan, capers, lemon zest and parsley as well as salt and a generous grind of black pepper. Place a

lid on the pan and leave to sit for 5 mins
before serving in deep bowls.

Eggy bread

Prep:5 mins

Cook:5 mins

Easy

Serves 1

The simplest of indulgent breakfast recipes.
Serve our eggy bread by itself, with an oozy fruit
compote or as part of a traditional fried
breakfast

Ingredients

- 2 medium eggs
- 1 tbsp milk
- 2 slices white bread or brown bread
- 1 tbsp butter

Method

1. Lightly beat the egg in a shallow bowl along with the milk. Season with salt and black pepper.

2. Dip each slice of bread into the egg mixture, making sure it has soaked up all of the liquid. Heat a frying pan over a medium heat and add the butter. Swirl the butter around the pan and when it's beginning to foam, add the bread and fry on each side for 1 min or until golden brown. Transfer to a plate and serve with crispy bacon or fruit compote.

Super sausage rolls

Prep:25 mins

Cook:35 mins

Plus cooling and chilling

Easy

Makes 12

Eat these family-friendly sausage rolls with a chutney or pickle. They make a great snack for a party buffet

Ingredients

- 375g all-butter puff pastry
- flour, for dusting
- tbsp apple sauce, pickle or chutney
- 400g sausagemeat or sausages, skins removed
- 1 egg, beaten
- tsp sesame seeds or nigella seeds (optional)

Method

1. Roll out the pastry to a 35 x 30cm rectangle on a surface lightly dusted with flour. Trim the edges neatly, then cut in half lengthways to form two long strips. Spread with a thin layer of the apple

sauce, pickle or chutney, leaving a border along the edges.

2. Tip the sausagemeat into a large bowl, add 3 tbsp cold water and squash together. Divide the mixture in two and mould each half into a cylindrical shape. Put each portion of meat into the middle of a pastry strip, leaving a border at either side. Brush the pastry border and the top of the sausage mix with the beaten egg. Fold one edge of the pastry over the meat and roll to encase, then use a fork to press the pastry edges together. Cut the sausage rolls into 5cm lengths and arrange on a lined baking tray. Chill for 20 mins. Can be made a day ahead or frozen for up to one month; to bake from frozen, add an extra 10 mins to the cooking time.

3. Heat oven to 200C/180C fan/gas 6. Brush the sausage rolls with the rest of the beaten egg and sprinkle with the sesame

seeds or nigella seeds (if using). Bake for
30-35 mins until the pastry is deep golden.
Transfer the sausage rolls to a wire rack
and leave to cool for 10 mins.

Prep:10 mins

Cook:30 mins

Easy

Serves 4

You'll need only five ingredients for this brunch-
friendly one-pan recipe- let paprika from the
sausage infuse the onion and new potatoes

Ingredients

- 500g baby new potato

- onions , sliced

- red peppers , deseeded and cut into strips

- 200g cooking chorizo , sliced

- eggs

Method

1. Steam the potatoes for 15-20 mins or until cooked.

2. Heat 1 tbsp oil in a non-stick pan. Add the onions and peppers, then cook for about 10 mins until soft. Push the peppers to the side of the pan and add the chorizo, sizzling until cooked though and releasing its oils. Transfer to a plate.

3. Once cool enough, halve the potatoes. Heat 1 tbsp oil in another non-stick pan and tip in the spuds. Fry for about 10 mins until golden and beginning to crisp. Stir in the onion mix, heat through and season.

4. Meanwhile, in the onion pan, fry the eggs to your liking. Place them on top of everything, allowing 1 egg per person.

Prep:10 mins

Cook:5 mins

Easy

Serves 1

Bring together two great brunch recipes – eggy bread and avocado on toast – then add a Mexican twist. A hit of chilli takes this to another level

Ingredients

- ½ medium ripe avocado , stoned and cut into pieces
- 2 medium tomatoes , deseeded and diced
- 1heaped tbsp chopped coriander
- ½ lime , juiced
- 2 large eggs , lightly beaten
- olive oil , for frying
- 2 thick slices sourdough or crusty bread
- 15g strong cheddar , grated

- ½ small red chilli , finely chopped

Method

2. Gently combine the avocado, tomato, coriander and lime juice in a small bowl. Season generously and set aside.

3. Whisk the eggs together with a little seasoning. Heat the oil in a non-stick frying pan over a medium heat. Dip each slice of bread in the egg mixture, coating well, then put the slices in the pan and cook for about 2 mins on each side or until golden brown. Put the eggy bread on a baking sheet, sprinkle with cheese and put under a hot grill for 1 min to melt. Top with the avocado salsa and red chilli to serve.

Bhaji burger

Prep:30 mins

Cook:20 mins

plus chilling

More effort

Serves 3

We've combined two of our favourite recipes to
make a bhaji in a bun. Serve with mango
chutney and a fluffy brioche bun

Ingredients

- For the burgers
- 400g lamb mince
- 2 tbsp tandoori paste
- 1 tsp cumin seeds
- For the raita
- ½ cucumber
- 150g pot plain yogurt
- ½ small pack mint , leaves chopped
- For the bhajis
- 100g plain flour
- 1 tbsp garam masala

- 1 tsp bicarbonate of soda

- 1 onion , halved and finely sliced

- 3 tbsp sunflower oil

- To serve

- 3 burger buns (we used brioche buns), toasted

- a few lettuce leaves

- red onion , thinly sliced

- mango chutney

Method

1. First, make the burgers. Tip all the ingredients into a bowl with a good pinch of salt and squeeze together with your fingers. Shape into three patties and chill in the fridge.

2. For the raita, grate the cucumber and squeeze out as much liquid as you can. Put in a bowl with the yogurt, mint and some salt. Mix and chill.

3. For the bhajis, tip the flour, spices and bicarb into a bowl with a pinch of salt. Slowly add 200ml cold water to make a thick batter (you might not need all of it), then mix in the onion.

4. Heat the oil in a large frying pan. Add the batter in batches so you have three burger-sized bhajis. Sizzle for 3 mins until crispy on one side, then flip and cook on the other side until cooked through. Keep warm.

5. Barbecue, griddle or pan-fry the burgers to your liking. Put lettuce and a burger on each bun and top with some raita, a bhaji and red onion. Serve the mango chutney on the side.

Carrot pilaf with coriander chutney

Prep:15 mins

Cook:35 mins

Easy

Serves 4

Try this healthy pilaf filled for an easy midweek meal. With cashew nuts, veg and spices, it's not only tasty but budget-friendly too. Top with coriander chutney

Ingredients

- tbsp rapeseed oil
- 1 large onion, finely sliced
- tbsp grated ginger
- green chillies, sliced
- garlic cloves, crushed
- tsp coriander seeds, crushed
- cardamom pods, bruised
- ½ cinnamon stick
- 1 tbsp garam masala
- 400g carrots, peeled and ½ coarsely grated, ½ sliced on an angle
- 300g basmati rice, rinsed well
- 600ml hot vegetable stock

- large bunch of coriander, finely chopped (stalks included)
- 60g cashews, toasted and chopped

Method

1. Heat the oil in a large pan that has a tight-fitting lid. Fry the onions with a pinch of salt over a medium heat for 10-15 mins until golden and crisp. Remove from the pan with a slotted spoon and drain on kitchen paper, leaving the oil in the pan.

2. Add half the ginger, half the chilli, all the garlic, spices, and both types of carrots to the pan, and fry for 6-8 mins until the carrot slices are starting to turn golden. Add the rice, stir briefly, then add the stock, a handful of the coriander, a good pinch of salt and grinding of black pepper. Bring to a simmer, and as soon as it starts to boil, turn the heat down to low,

cover with a lid and leave to cook for 12-15 mins.

3. Meanwhile, put the remaining ginger and green chilli, most of the cashews and most of the remaining coriander in a small blender with 50ml water. Blend until smooth, adding another 2-3 tbsp water, if needed, to make a spoonable sauce.

4. When all the liquid has been absorbed into the pilaf and the rice is tender, fluff up the grains with a fork. Spoon over the coriander chutney, and sprinkle with the fried onions, reserved coriander and remaining cashews to serve.

Easy millionaire's shortbread

Prep:25 mins

Cook:35 mins

Easy

Makes up to 24 squares

Combine the crunch of a shortbread base with a gooey caramel middle and chocolate topping, and you have millionaire's shortbread – the ultimate sweet treat

Ingredients

- For the shortbread
- 250g plain flour
- 75g caster sugar
- 175g butter, softened

- For the caramel
- 100g butter or margarine
- 100g light muscovado sugar
- 397g can condensed milk
- For the topping
- 200g plain or milk chocolate, broken into pieces

Method

1. Heat the oven to 180C/160C fan/gas 4. Lightly grease and line a 20-22cm square or rectangular baking tin with a lip of at least 3cm.

2. To make the shortbread, mix 250g plain flour and 75g caster sugar in a bowl. Rub in 175g softened butter until the mixture resembles fine breadcrumbs.

3. Knead the mixture together until it forms a dough, then press into the base of the prepared tin.

4. Prick the shortbread lightly with a fork and bake for 20 minutes or until firm to the touch and very lightly browned. Leave to cool in the tin.

5. To make the caramel, place 100g butter or margarine, 100g light muscovado sugar and the can of condensed milk in a pan and heat gently until the sugar has

dissolved. Continually stir with a spatula
to make sure no sugar sticks to the
bottom of the pan. (This can leave brown
specks in the caramel but won't affect the
flavour.)

6. Turn up the heat to medium high, stirring
   all the time, and bring to the boil, then
   lower the heat back to low and stirring
   continuously, for about 5-10 minutes or
   until the mixture has thickened slightly.
   Pour over the shortbread and leave to
   cool.

7. For the topping, melt 200g plain or milk
   chocolate slowly in a bowl over a pan of
   hot water. Pour over the cold caramel and
   leave to set. Cut into squares or bars with
   a hot knife.

Orzo & tomato soup

Prep:5 mins

Cook:25 mins

Easy

Serves 4

Make our simple, budget-friendly tomato, orzo and chickpea soup in just 30 minutes. This easy, vegetarian family meal is healthy and even low fat

Ingredients

- tbsp olive oil
- 1 onion, chopped
- celery sticks, chopped
- garlic cloves, crushed
- 1 tbsp tomato purée
- 400g can chopped tomatoes
- 400g can chickpeas
- 150g orzo pasta
- 700ml vegetable stock
- 2 tbsp basil pesto
- crusty bread, to serve

Method

Heat 1 tbsp olive oil in a large saucepan. Add the onion and celery and fry for 10-15 mins, or until starting to soften, then add the garlic and cook for 1 min more. Stir in all the other ingredients, except for the pesto and remaining oil, and bring to the boil.

Reduce the heat and leave to simmer for 6-8 mins, or until the orzo is tender. Season to taste, then ladle into bowls.

Stir the remaining oil with the pesto, then drizzle over the soup. Serve with chunks of crusty bread.

Spiced lamb kebabs with pea & herb couscous

Prep:20 mins

Cook:20 mins

Easy

Makes 6 skewers, 2 per adult, 1 per child

These peppery paprika lamb skewers are barbecue friendly. Serve with a vegetable couscous flavoured with mint and coriander

Ingredients

- 400g lean lamb shoulder, cut into 3cm cubes
- 1 tsp ground cumin
- ½ tsp cayenne pepper
- 1 tsp sweet smoked paprika
- 1 tbsp olive oil
- 24 cherry tomatoes
- 140g couscous
- 400ml hot vegetable stock
- 140g frozen pea
- 1 large carrot , coarsely grated
- small pack coriander , chopped
- small pack mint , chopped
- juice 1 lemon
- tbsp extra virgin olive oil

Method

1. Soak 6 wooden skewers in water for 30
    mins (this prevents them burning when
    cooking on the griddle or barbecue). Put
    the lamb cubes in a large bowl with the
    spices and olive oil. Toss everything
    together well and season.
2. Thread a piece of lamb onto a skewer,
    followed by a cherry tomato. Repeat,
    adding about 4 pieces of lamb and 4
    cherry tomatoes to each skewer, until all
    are used up.
3. Meanwhile, put the couscous in a large
    bowl, pour over the hot vegetable stock
    and add the peas. Stir, then cover with
    cling film and leave to soak, about 5 mins.
4. Heat a griddle pan. When all the liquid
    has soaked into the couscous, gently fluff
    up the grains using a fork, and stir in the
    carrot, herbs, lemon juice and olive oil.
    Mix everything together well, season and
    set aside.

5. Place the skewers on the hot griddle pan and cook for 5-6 mins, then turn and cook for a further 5-6 mins until the meat and tomatoes are charred and cooked through. Serve the skewers with the couscous.

Puttanesca baked gnocchi

Prep:5 mins

Cook:30 mins

Easy

Serves 4

Serve this budget-friendly baked gnocchi with tomatoes, mozzarella, capers and olives for a delicious midweek family meal when you're short on time

Ingredients

- x 400g cans cherry tomatoes
- olive oil, for frying

- 1 onion, finely chopped

- 1 tsp chilli flakes

- 1 tbsp capers, drained

- 60g black pitted Kalamata olives, roughly chopped

- anchovy fillets in oil, finely chopped

- pinch of sugar

- 500g shop-bought gnocchi

- 1 x 125g ball mozzarella, torn

Method

1. Blitz one of the cans of tomatoes until smooth and set aside. Heat a glug of oil in a medium-sized saucepan over a medium heat. Add the onion and a generous pinch of salt and fry gently for 8-10 mins until softened and translucent. Tip the chilli and all the tomatoes into the pan, lower the heat, then simmer for 10 mins, uncovered. Fill one of the empty cans a quarter full with water and add this to the

sauce. Stir through the capers, olives and
anchovies. Season with salt, pepper and a
couple of generous pinches of sugar.
Cook on a gentle heat, uncovered, for a
further 5 mins. Keep warm until needed.

2. Bring a large pan of water to the boil.
Add the gnocchi and cook for 2 mins.
Drain and toss with the tomato sauce,
then tip into an ovenproof dish or
shallow casserole. Top with the torn
mozzarella and a good grating of black
pepper then pop under a high grill for 3-4
mins or until the mozzarella is molten
and gooey.

Curried kale & chickpea soup

Prep:10 mins

Cook:25 mins

Easy

Serves 2

Rustle up this budget-friendly, healthy soup for a nourishing, easy midweek meal. It's packed with kale, chickpeas, sweet potato and plenty of flavour

Ingredients

- 1 tsp rapeseed or coconut oil
- 1 onion, chopped
- 1 tbsp grated ginger
- garlic cloves, crushed
- 1 sweet potato (about 200g), peeled and cut into 2cm cubes
- 1 tsp turmeric
- tsp ground cumin
- tbsp medium or hot curry powder
- 400g can chickpeas, rinsed
- 150ml low-fat coconut milk
- 500ml vegetable stock (see tip, below)
- 160g kale, chopped
- 1 lime, juiced
- 1 red chilli, finely chopped (optional)

Method

1. Heat the oil in a large pan and fry the onion for 5 mins. Add the ginger and garlic, fry for 1 min more, then stir in the sweet potato, spices and chickpeas. Cook for another 5 mins, adding a little water if the spices stick to the pan.

2. Pour in the coconut milk and 400ml of the stock, then bring to a simmer and cook for 8 mins. Season, then transfer a quarter of the soup to a blender and whizz until smooth. Pour in the reserved stock to loosen, if needed, then add back to the pan with the remaining soup. Stir in the kale and cook for 5 mins. Add the lime juice, then ladle into bowls and scatter over the chilli, if you like.

RECIPE TIPS

CREAMY TWIST

For a creamier soup, swap 250ml of the vegetable stock for another 250ml coconut milk.

Prep:5 mins

Cook:30 mins

Easy

Serves 4

Take your stew or casserole to the next level with our easy dumplings. Add them to your dish for instant family-friendly comfort food in a flash

Ingredients

- 150g self-raising flour, plus a little extra
- 70g suet
- small handful of parsley, chopped (optional)

Method

1. Whilst your stew is bubbling, make the dumplings. Weigh the flour into a bowl and add ½ tsp salt. Stir through the suet and parsley, if using. Make a well in the centre and add 3 tbsp cold water, mix to a dough, adding more water until the dough is firm but pliable. Divide into eight equal pieces and roll in a little more flour into balls. Chill until needed.

2. When the stew has about 30 mins to go, arrange the dumplings on top and cover with a lid. With the oven at 160C/140C fan/gas 3, cook the stew and dumplings for 20 mins, then remove the lid and cook for another 10 mins until they're brown and puffed up.

Easy millionaire's shortbread

Prep:25 mins

Cook:35 mins

Easy

Makes up to 24 squares

Combine the crunch of a shortbread base with a gooey caramel middle and chocolate topping, and you have millionaire's shortbread – the ultimate sweet treat

Ingredients

- For the shortbread
- 250g plain flour
- 75g caster sugar
- 175g butter, softened
- For the caramel
- 100g butter or margarine
- 100g light muscovado sugar
- 397g can condensed milk
- For the topping
- 200g plain or milk chocolate, broken into pieces

Method

1. Heat the oven to 180C/160C fan/gas 4. Lightly grease and line a 20-22cm square or rectangular baking tin with a lip of at least 3cm.

2. To make the shortbread, mix 250g plain flour and 75g caster sugar in a bowl. Rub in 175g softened butter until the mixture resembles fine breadcrumbs.

3. Knead the mixture together until it forms a dough, then press into the base of the prepared tin.

4. Prick the shortbread lightly with a fork and bake for 20 minutes or until firm to the touch and very lightly browned. Leave to cool in the tin.

5. To make the caramel, place 100g butter or margarine, 100g light muscovado sugar and the can of condensed milk in a pan and heat gently until the sugar has dissolved. Continually stir with a spatula to make sure no sugar sticks to the

bottom of the pan. (This can leave brown specks in the caramel but won't affect the flavour.)

6. Turn up the heat to medium high, stirring all the time, and bring to the boil, then lower the heat back to low and stirring continuously, for about 5-10 minutes or until the mixture has thickened slightly. Pour over the shortbread and leave to cool.

7. For the topping, melt 200g plain or milk chocolate slowly in a bowl over a pan of hot water. Pour over the cold caramel and leave to set. Cut into squares or bars with a hot knife.

Spinach & ricotta pancake bake

Prep:10 mins

Cook:35 mins

Easy

Serves 4

Make pancakes on Shrove Tuesday and serve
our spinach and ricotta pancake bake for dinner.
For dessert, choose one of our sweet pancake
recipes

Ingredients

- 1 tbsp olive oil , plus a drizzle
- 3 garlic cloves , crushed
- 400g can chopped tomatoes
- 200g bag baby spinach
- 250g tub ricotta
- grating of nutmeg
- 4 large pancakes or crêpes (see recipe, below)
- 225g ball mozzarella , drained and torn into small pieces
- 50g parmesan or vegetarian alternative, grated

Method

1. Heat the oil in a pan, add 2 garlic cloves
   and sizzle for a few seconds, then tip in
   the tomatoes. Season, and bubble for 10-
   15 mins until reduced to a thick sauce.
   Microwave the spinach for 2 mins to wilt,
   or by tipping into a colander and pouring
   over a kettle full of hot water. When cool
   enough to handle, squeeze out as much
   liquid as you can, then roughly chop.

2. Heat the oven to 220C/200C fan/gas 7.
   Mix together the ricotta, spinach, a
   generous grating of nutmeg, the
   remaining crushed garlic and some salt
   and pepper. Spread the tomato sauce over
   the base of a shallow baking dish about
   20cm x 30cm. Divide the spinach mixture
   between the pancakes, spreading it over
   half the surface. Fold each pancake in
   half, then in half again to make a triangle.
   Lay the pancakes on top of the sauce,
   scatter with the mozzarella and

parmesan. Drizzle with a little more oil and bake for 15-20 mins until bubbling.

Speedy sausage stroganoff tagliatelle

Prep:5 mins

Cook:15 mins

Easy

Serves 4

Make our budget-friendly quick sausage stroganoff tagliatelle for a simple family dinner. This filling bowl takes just five minutes to prepare

Ingredients

- 20g unsalted butter
- olive oil, for drizzling
- pork sausages
- 350g chestnut mushrooms, sliced
- 1 tsp sweet smoked paprika
- 300ml soured cream

- ½ tbsp wholegrain mustard

- 150ml beef stock

- 400g dried tagliatelle

- small bunch parsley, chopped

Method

1. Heat the butter and oil in a frying pan over a medium-high heat until foaming. Squeeze large chunks of the sausagemeat out of the skins and into the pan. Cook for 5-8 mins or until golden brown. Add the mushrooms and cook for a further 5 mins until starting to turn brown. Stir through the paprika and cook for 1 min before stirring in the soured cream, mustard and stock. Bring to a simmer and season to taste.

2. Meanwhile, cook the pasta in a large pan of salted water according to pack instructions, then add to the sauce with

half the parsley. Serve in deep bowls with
the remaining parsley sprinkled on top.

Prep:10 mins

Cook:55 mins

Easy

Serves 4

Enjoy the spicy, rich flavours of tikka masala
with this family-friendly lighter version that's
both healthy and gluten-free. It's a guaranteed
crowd-pleaser

Ingredients

- 1 large onion , chopped
- large garlic cloves
- thumb-sized piece of ginger
- tbsp rapeseed oil

- small skinless chicken breasts, cut into chunks
- tbsp tikka spice powder
- 1 tsp cayenne pepper
- 400g can chopped tomatoes
- 40g ground almonds
- 200g spinach
- tbsp fat-free natural yogurt
- ½ small bunch of coriander , chopped
- brown basmati rice , to serve

Method

1. Put the onion, garlic and ginger in a food processor and whizz to a smooth paste.

2. Heat 1 tbsp of the oil in a flameproof casserole dish over a medium heat. Add the onion mixture and fry for 15 mins. Tip into a bowl and wipe out the pan.

3. Add the remaining oil and the chicken and fry for 5-7 mins, or until lightly brown. Stir in the tikka spice and cayenne

and fry for a further minute. Tip the onion mixture back into the pan, along with the tomatoes and 1 can full of water. Bring to the boil, then reduce to a simmer and cook, uncovered, for 15 mins. Stir in the almonds and spinach and cook for a further 10 mins. Season, then stir though the yogurt and coriander. Serve with brown rice.

Crusty cheddar pies

Prep:20 mins

Cook:1 hr and 25 mins

Easy

Makes 8 individual pies

This recipe has been designed to be made ahead and frozen - a family-friendly batch pie, with cheesy mashed potato atop hidden broccoli, leeks and celery

Ingredients

- 500g slim young leek , thickly sliced

- 300g broccoli , cut into small florets

- celery sticks, de-stringed and sliced

- 1 ½kg floury potato , such as King Edward, cut into even-sized chunks

- 85g butter

- 170g pot 0% fat Greek yogurt

- 850ml semi-skimmed milk

- 75g plain flour

- tsp English mustard

- 1 tsp wholegrain mustard

- 300g pack mature cheddar , finely grated

- handful frozen peas

Method

1. Bring a large pan of salted water to the boil. Put the leeks, broccoli and celery in a large steamer. Add the potatoes to the water and cook for 20 mins, with the vegetables steaming on top, until all are

tender. Drain the potatoes, then mash with plenty of seasoning, 25g of the butter and all the yogurt.

2. While the veg cooks, pour the milk into a pan, add the flour, both mustards and remaining butter, and cook over a medium heat, whisking all the time, until smooth and thickened. Stir in half the cheese and season. Remove from heat.

3. Divide the steamed veg and peas between 8 individual pie dishes. Pour over the sauce and top with the mash, then sprinkle over the remaining cheese.

4. Pack into freezer bags and use within 3 months. To serve, unwrap and put the dishes on a baking tray in the cold oven, then set to 200C/180C fan/ gas 6. Bake for 50-55 mins until bubbling and hot all the way through.

RECIPE TIPS

COOKING FROM FRESH

If you want to cook this dish straightaway. Pop it in a preheated oven for 25 mins instead of freezing.

Spiced red lentil soup

Prep:5 mins

Cook:30 mins

Easy

Serves 4 - 6

Simple soups like this make great lunches - and are wallet-friendly too!

Ingredients

- 1 onion , chopped
- 1 tbsp olive oil
- 1-2 tbsp Thai red curry paste
- 300g red lentil
- 1.7l vegetable stock
- 200ml coconut milk

- chopped spring onions , to serve (optional)

Method

1. Fry the onion in 1 tbsp olive oil until soft. Stir in the red Thai curry paste, depending how hot you want it.

2. Add red lentils and mix to coat in the paste. Pour over vegetable stock and simmer for 20 mins until the lentils are tender.

3. Blend with coconut milk and reheat if needed. Serve scattered with chopped spring onions, if you like.

Pesto salmon & bean gratins

Prep:15 mins

Cook:20 mins

Easy

Serves 6

Keep everyone in the family happy with our freezer-friendly seafood bake. You can freeze individual portions – just remember to label them with the cooking instructions

Ingredients

- 100g baby spinach
- x 400g cans cannellini beans , drained
- 300g cherry tomatoes , halved
- tbsp olive oil
- 1 lemon , zested and juiced
- tbsp soft cheese
- tbsp pesto
- 150g breadcrumbs
- 40g parmesan , grated
- tbsp pine nuts
- salmon fillets, skin removed
- crusty bread , to serve (optional)

Method

1. Divide the spinach between six individual
    baking dishes (make sure the dishes are
    safe to use from the freezer to the oven).
    Spoon over the beans and tomatoes and
    drizzle with the oil. Scatter over a little of
    the lemon zest and squeeze over some
    juice, then season well. Toss everything
    together with your hands, like you would
    a salad.

2. Mix the soft cheese and pesto together in
    one bowl, and the breadcrumbs,
    parmesan and pine nuts in another.
    Season the salmon fillets and lay one in
    each dish, then spread the soft cheese mix
    over the fillets. Scatter with the cheesy
    breadcrumbs, pressing onto the salmon
    (it's okay if it also gets on the veg and
    beans a little).

3. If you want to cook straightaway, heat the
    oven to 200C/180C fan/gas 6 and bake for

20-25 mins, or until the salmon is cooked through and the crumbs are golden.

4. Alternatively, cover the dishes well and freeze for up to two months – it's a good idea to write the name of the dish and the cooking instructions on the lid. To cook from frozen, uncover and bake for 30-35 mins at 200C/180C fan/gas 6.

5. Serve the gratins with some crusty bread for mopping up the juices, if you like.

Slow-cooker sausage casserole

Prep:20 mins

Cook:4 hrs

4 hrs on high or 8 hrs on low

Easy

Serves 4

You can use your favourite type of sausages to make this family-friendly slow-cooker casserole.

Serve it over pasta, in baked potatoes or with bread

Ingredients

- red onions , finely chopped
- 1 celery stick , finely chopped
- 1-2 tbsp rapeseed oil
- carrots , cut into fat pieces
- 12 chipolatas , each halved
- 1 sweet potato , peeled and cut into chunks
- 400g tin tomatoes
- 1 tbsp tomato purée or tomato and veg purée
- 1 thyme sprig
- 1 rosemary sprig
- 1 beef stock cube or stock pot

Method

1. Fry the onion and celery in the oil over a low heat until it starts to soften and cook,

about 5 mins, then spoon it into the slow cooker. Fry the carrots briefly and add them too.

2. Brown the sausages all over in the same frying pan – make sure they get a really good colour because they won't get any browner in the slow cooker. Transfer to the slow cooker and add the sweet potato and tomatoes.

3. Put the purée in the frying pan and add 250ml boiling water, swirl everything around to pick up every last bit of flavour, and tip the lot into the slow cooker. Add the herbs, stock cube and some pepper. Don't add salt until the casserole is cooked as the stock can be quite salty. Cook on high for 4 hrs or on low for 8 hrs, then serve or leave to cool and freeze.

RECIPE TIPS

SLOW COOKERS

Slow cookers vary in capacity and efficiency –
you may want to check casserole timings against
the manufacturers' instructions on yours.

Lemony prawn & chorizo rice pot

Prep:15 mins

Cook:25 mins

Easy

Serves 4

Spanish classic paella is given a healthy
makeover and a good kick of heat - diet-friendly
and fresh

Ingredients

- 1 tbsp olive oil
- 1 onion , sliced
- small red peppers , deseeded and sliced
- 50g chorizo , thinly sliced
- garlic cloves , crushed

- 1 red chilli (deseeded if you don't like it too hot)
- ½ tsp turmeric
- 250g long grain rice
- 200g raw peeled prawn , defrosted if frozen
- 100g frozen pea
- zest and juice 1 lemon , plus extra wedges to serve

Method

1. Boil the kettle. Heat the oil in a shallow pan with a lid, add the onion, peppers, chorizo, garlic and chilli, then fry over a high heat for 3 mins. Add the turmeric and rice, stirring to ensure the rice is coated. Pour in 500ml boiling water, cover, then cook for 12 mins.

2. Uncover, then stir – the rice should be almost tender. Stir in the prawns and peas, with a splash more water if the rice

is looking dry, then cook for 1 min more until the prawns are just pink and the rice tender. Stir in the lemon zest and juice with seasoning and serve with extra lemon wedges on the side.

RECIPE TIPS

OVEN-BAKING

1. If you don't want to spend time at the stove, you can bake this dish in the oven. Tip the oil, onion, peppers, chorizo, garlic and chilli into an ovenproof dish, then bake for 15 mins at 200C/180C fan/gas 6. Stir in the turmeric, rice and water, cover, then bake for another 20 mins, stirring in prawns and peas for the final 2 mins. Season and stir in lemon zest and juice to serve.

Cheesy scrambled egg croissants

Prep:5 mins

Cook:5 mins

Easy

Serves 4

These breakfast baps with creamy eggs are camping-friendly, but work just as well as a casual brunch

Ingredients

- large eggs
- 100g grated cheddar
- a splash of milk
- small bunch chives , snipped
- large croissants

Method

1. In a bowl, whisk the eggs, cheddar, milk and some seasoning. Pour into a saucepan and heat gently, stirring continuously, until softly scrambled. Stir in chives, then split open croissants

(warm them first if you have an oven) and put the scrambled eggs inside.

Chipotle sweet potato & black bean stew with cheddar dumplings

Prep:10 mins

Cook:50 mins

Easy

Serves 4

Enjoy this filling sweet potato and black bean stew as a budget-friendly midweek meal. Served with moreish cheddar dumplings, it's great for feeding a crowd

Ingredients

- vegetable oil , for frying
- 1 large red onion , finely sliced
- 250g bag diced butternut squash and sweet potato
- 400g can chopped tomatoes

- x 400g cans chilli black beans or chilli kidney beans
- tbsp chipotle chilli paste
- 125g self-raising flour
- 60g unsalted butter , cubed
- 70g mature cheddar , grated
- 1 large green jalapeño , finely sliced (optional)

Method

1. Heat a glug of vegetable oil in a large flameproof casserole over a medium heat. Add the onion and a pinch of salt and cook for 7 mins until softened. Tip in the squash and sweet potato and fry for a few minutes before adding the tomatoes, beans and 250ml water. Stir through the chipotle paste and season to taste. Pop a lid on the dish and gently simmer over a low to medium heat for 25 mins or until reduced and the sweet potato is soft.

2. Heat the oven to 200C/180C fan/ gas 6.
    Mix the flour with ½ tsp salt. Add the
    butter and rub together with your fingers
    until the mixture resembles fine
    breadcrumbs. Stir in the grated cheddar
    then quickly mix in 4 tbsp cold water. Roll
    the mixture into eight balls. Put the
    dumplings on top of the stew and place,
    uncovered, in the oven for 15-20 mins, or
    until puffed up and light golden brown.
    Serve the stew with the sliced jalapeño
    scattered on top, if you like.

Chicken & bacon cacciatore

Prep:30 mins

Cook:1 hr and 15 mins

Easy

Serves 4 - 6

By using a whole chicken and freezing leftovers
this tasty supper is extra penny-friendly

Ingredients

- tbsp olive oil

- 1 large chicken , roughly 1.8kg-2.2kg, jointed into 8 pieces

- rashers streaky bacon , chopped

- onions , sliced

- rosemary sprigs

- x cans plum tomatoes

- tbsp red or white wine vinegar

- 1 tbsp sugar

- 500ml chicken stock

- small bunch parsley , chopped (optional)

Method

1. Heat the oil in a large casserole dish. Brown the chicken, a few pieces at a time, until skin is golden on all sides. As each piece is done, lift out onto a plate. Turn the heat down and add the bacon. Cook gently so some of the fat melts into the pan and keep going until the bacon

crisps. Lift out with a slotted spoon and put with the chicken pieces, then add the onions and rosemary to the casserole. Fry for 5-10 mins until the onions have softened, then return the chicken and bacon, along with the tomatoes, vinegar, sugar, stock and seasoning.

2. Bring to a simmer, cover and cook for 40-50 mins until the chicken is tender – check one of the thigh or leg joints as they will take longer to cook. Stir in the parsley, if using, check the seasoning again and serve with mash, pasta or rice if eating straight away. Otherwise, cool and chill for up to 24 hrs. Or freeze for up to 3 months. Defrost overnight in the fridge, then bring out to room temperature the next day if not fully defrosted. Tip back into a saucepan, bring to a gentle simmer, then cover and gently cook until chicken

is piping hot. Don't boil or the chicken may toughen up.

Prep:10 mins

Cook:1 hr and 15 mins

Easy

Serves 1

The perfect budget-friendly, filling supper for one. The fragrant, zesty flavour of sumac is a refreshing contrast to the creamy whipped feta

Ingredients

- 1 baking potato
- tsp olive oil
- ½ tsp garlic salt
- 50g feta
- 50g Greek yogurt

- 1 roasted red peppers from a jar (about 25g), finely chopped
- ½ tsp sumac
- few basil leaves , to serve (optional)

Method

1. Heat oven to 220C/200C fan/ gas 6. Prick the potato all over with a fork and bake for 1 hr until it is golden outside and soft inside. Mix 1 tsp olive oil with the garlic salt. Cut a deep cross into the top of the jacket, drizzle the garlic oil into the cross and rub it all over the outside. Return to the oven and bake for 15 mins more until the edges are golden and crispy.

2. Meanwhile, crumble the feta into a bowl, add the yogurt and whisk together until creamy. Stir in the red pepper with a good grind of black pepper and spoon the whipped feta into the jacket. Sprinkle with the sumac, drizzle over the

remaining 1 tsp olive oil and scatter a few torn basil leaves on top, if you like.

Prep:15 mins

Cook:35 mins

Easy

Serves 6

Whip up this warming, family-friendly dessert in under an hour using apples and golden caramel. Serve hot from the oven with a scoop of ice cream

Ingredients

- 1 tbsp butter, softened
- large eggs, and 2 egg yolks
- 50g dark brown soft sugar
- 200ml whole milk
- 300ml double cream
- 375g can caramel, beaten until smooth

- tsp vanilla extract

- 75g plain flour

- apples (we used Pink Lady)

- ice cream, to serve (optional)

Method

1. Heat the oven to 180C/160C fan/gas 4.
   Butter a 30 x 20 x 4cm baking dish. Put the
   eggs, extra yolks, sugar, milk, cream, 200g
   of the caramel, the vanilla and a large
   pinch of sea salt in a large bowl, then
   whisk until combined. Stir in the flour
   until the batter is smooth.

2. Halve, core and cut the apples into 1cm
   slices – there's no need to peel them.
   Arrange in the baking dish and pour over
   the batter. Bake for 30-35 mins until the
   batter is set in the centre, golden and
   slightly risen.

3. Drizzle over the remaining caramel, then
   sprinkle with a little extra sea salt. Leave

to rest for 5-10 mins (it will deflate a little). Serve warm with vanilla or peanut butter ice cream, if you like.

RECIPE TIPS

If you prefer a little less sweetness in your dessert, go for a sharper apple variety like Cox or Russet.

Child-friendly Thai chicken noodles

Prep:10 mins

Cook:15 mins - 20 mins

Easy

Serves 2 adults + 2 children

Introduce exotic flavours to your kids with this subtly spiced, fragrant Thai chicken curry. Make it in 30 minutes and refrigerate leftovers for tomorrow's lunch

Ingredients

- 100g sugar snap peas

- 1 tbsp oil

- 2 spring onions , finely chopped

- 2 garlic cloves , crushed

- 1 tsp grated ginger

- 3 x chicken breasts, cut into chunks

- ½ tbsp Thai curry paste (we used Thai Taste)

- 400ml can coconut milk

- limes , juice of one, other quartered

- 50g frozen peas

- nests egg noodles

- handful chopped coriander , to serve

Method

1. Blanch the sugar snap peas in a bowl of boiling water for 2 mins, then drain. Heat the oil in a large frying pan. Add the spring onions, garlic, ginger and chicken. Gently fry for 2-3 mins. Stir in the curry paste and cook for 1 minute more. Add the coconut milk to the pan, along with a

splash of water, the lime juice, peas and
sugar snap peas. Gently bubble for
around 5 mins until the chicken is cooked
through.

2. Meanwhile, cook the noodles according
to the pack instructions. Drain. Stir the
noodles through the sauce, scatter with
coriander and serve with a wedge of lime
for squeezing over.

Prep:20 mins

Cook:5 mins - 10 mins

plus 1 hr marinating

Easy

Serves 4

Make these family-friendly chicken wraps with
lemon, garlic and cinnamon marinade on a
barbecue if the sun is shining. Serve in flatbreads
with yoghurt

Ingredients

- skinless chicken breasts , cut into strips
- 1 lemon
- 1 tsp dried oregano (optional)
- 1 garlic clove , crushed
- pinch of cinnamon
- 1 tbsp olive oil
- flatbreads
- tbsp Greek yogurt
- ¼ red pepper , finely chopped
- 1 Little Gem lettuce , finely chopped

Method

1. Put the chicken in a bowl. Pare strips of zest from the lemon using a vegetable peeler, then juice the lemon too. Add the peel and half the juice to the chicken, along with the oregano (if using), garlic, cinnamon and oil. Mix well, cover and chill for an hour. The lemon juice will

start to 'cook' the chicken, so don't leave for longer.

2. Heat the barbecue. If you are using coals, wait until they turn white. If you are indoors, heat a griddle pan. Thread the chicken strips onto a couple of metal skewers to stop them falling through the grate (you don't need to do this for the griddle), then grill for a couple of mins each side. The strips will cook through quickly so don't leave them too long. Season if you like.

3. Warm the flatbreads on the edge of the barbecue (or on the griddle) for a minute, then transfer them to plates and spread each with ½ tbsp yogurt. Divide the chicken strips between them, then dot on the remaining yogurt and sprinkle over the pepper and lettuce. Fold or roll the flatbreads to eat.

Prep:35 mins

Cook:40 mins

Easy

Serves 6

This freezable, family-friendly recipe is economical and has a wonderful comfort-food feel about it

Ingredients

- large onions , halved and thinly sliced
- tbsp olive oil
- 1 tsp dried oregano
- 300g pack lean smoked back bacon , chopped
- x 400g cans chopped tomatoes in rich juice
- 20 basil leaves , roughly torn, plus extra to serve if you like

- 250g pack fresh egg lasagne (check pack for cooking instructions)
- For the white sauce
- 600ml milk
- 50g each butter and plain flour
- generous grating fresh nutmeg
- 50g grated parmesan

Method

1. Fry the onions in the oil for about 15 mins until golden. Add the oregano and bacon and fry for 5 mins more, stirring frequently. Tip in the tomatoes, season and bubble uncovered for 5 mins. Remove from the heat and stir in the basil.

2. Meanwhile, make the white sauce. Pour the milk into a pan and tip in the butter and flour. Whisk continuously over a moderate heat to incorporate the flour,

then simmer, stirring until thickened. Season with salt, pepper and nutmeg.

3. Spoon a third of the tomato sauce on the base of a lasagne dish. Top with a third of the lasagne sheets. Then top with a third sauce, a third lasagne, the last of the tomato sauce and finally the last sheets of lasagne. Pour over the white sauce and scatter with the cheese and an extra grating of nutmeg. Chill. If eating straight away, bake at 190C/170C fan/gas 5 for 40 mins until golden and bubbling. Scatter with basil, if you like, and serve with a salad and garlic bread.

4. To freeze, cool completely, then wrap in cling film, then foil. Will store for 3 months. To serve, thaw for 6 hrs in a cool place. Unwrap and bake at 190C/170C fan/gas 5 for 50-60 mins until thoroughly heated through.

Greek loaded fries

Prep:10 mins

Cook:15 mins

Easy

Serves 4 as a side

Bake some budget-friendly frozen fries and pile them high with a moreish Greek-inspired topping of feta, olives, tomatoes and cucumber. Great for sharing

Ingredients

- 400g frozen French fries
- 1 tsp dried oregano
- tsp olive oil
- ¼ finely chopped cucumber
- 10 pitted and halved black olives
- finely chopped cherry tomatoes
- 1 tbsp finely chopped parsley
- tbsp Greek yogurt
- 40g crumbled feta

Method

1. Toss the French fries with the dried oregano and olive oil, then cook following pack instructions.

2. While the fries are cooking, mix the cucumber with the black olives, cherry tomatoes and parsley. Mix the Greek yogurt with half of the crumbled feta in a separate bowl. Tip the fries into a serving dish, top with the salad and yogurt mixture, then scatter over the remaining crumbled feta. Season and serve.

Ginger, sesame and chilli prawn & broccoli stir-fry

Prep:5 mins

Cook:10 mins

Easy

Serves 2

Make our budget-friendly stir-fry with ginger, sesame and chilli prawns for a super-simple midweek meal. This speedy, low-fat supper makes a great dinner for two

Ingredients

- 250g broccoli , thin-stemmed if you like, cut into even-sized florets
- balls stem ginger , finely chopped, plus 2 tbsp syrup from the jar
- tbsp low-salt soy sauce
- 1 garlic clove , crushed
- 1 red chilli , a little thinly sliced, the rest deseeded and finely chopped
- tsp sesame seeds
- ½ tbsp sesame oil
- 200g raw king prawns
- 100g beansprouts
- cooked rice or noodles, to serve

Method

1. Heat a pan of water until boiling. Tip in
    the broccoli and cook for just 1 min – it
    should still have a good crunch.
    Meanwhile, mix the stem ginger and
    syrup, soy sauce, garlic and finely
    chopped chilli.

2. Toast the sesame seeds in a dry wok or
    large frying pan. When they're nicely
    browned, turn up the heat and add the
    oil, prawns and cooked broccoli. Stir-fry
    for a few mins until the prawns turn pink.
    Pour over the ginger sauce, then tip in the
    beansprouts. Cook for 30 seconds, or until
    the beansprouts are heated thoroughly,
    adding a splash more soy or ginger syrup,
    if you like. Scatter with the sliced chilli
    and serve over rice or noodles.

Open rye sandwich with halloumi & avocado

Prep:5 mins

No cook

Easy

Serves 2

A lunch-friendly rye bread sandwich with salty cheese and guacamole. Serve with a zesty squeeze of lime

Ingredients

- tbsp guacamole (from Cajun grilled halloumi, see 'goes well with')
- slices rye bread
- tomatoes , each sliced into 4
- slices (125g) Cajun-coated halloumi cheese (from Cajun gilled halloumi, see 'goes well with')
- squeeze of lime

Method

1. Heat the grill. Line a grill pan with foil and place the halloumi slices on it and grill for 3-4 mins, checking occasionally until golden.

2. Divide the guacamole between the 2 slices
    rye bread, spreading it evenly. Arrange 4
    slices of tomato on each sandwich, and
    top with the Cajun grilled halloumi slices.
    Finish with a squeeze of lime and some
    ground black pepper.

Cod with butter bean colcannon

Prep:5 mins

Cook:10 mins

Easy

Serves 2

Whip up a budget-friendly fish dinner with
creamy butter bean colcannon. It's the perfect
midweek meal for two and ready in just 15
minutes

Ingredients

- skinless cod fillets
- 25g butter

- thyme sprigs , leaves picked

- ½ lemon , sliced

- 77g pack smoked diced pancetta

- ½ small Savoy cabbage , finely shredded

- 400g can butter beans , drained and rinsed

- 50ml single cream

Method

1. Heat oven to 220C/200C fan/gas 8. Cut two squares of baking parchment slightly bigger than the cod and place a fillet in the centre of each one. Divide 20g of the butter between the two fillets and top with a few thyme leaves and lemon slices. Season generously. Fold and scrunch the paper together to create two paper parcels. Put on a baking sheet and cook for 8-10 mins.

2. Meanwhile, heat a medium-sized frying pan over a high heat and fry the pancetta

for a few mins until golden and crisp.
Add the remaining butter and cabbage,
then cook for 5 mins or until the cabbage
has softened. In a small saucepan over a
low heat, lightly mash the butter beans
with a potato masher, then mix the beans
through the buttery cabbage and pancetta
mixture. Stir through the cream to loosen
and season generously. Serve the fish
with the creamy colcannon.

Cowboy chicken & bean stew

Prep:10 mins

Cook:1 hr and 20 mins

Easy

Serves 4

A paprika-spiced casserole that's campsite-
friendly and warming for the tum- pinto beans
stretch the dish a little further

Ingredients

- drizzle of oil

- 1 large onion , chopped

- rashers smoked streaky bacon , chopped

- 8 chicken portions (we used thighs and drumsticks), skin removed

- 1 tbsp smoked paprika

- x 400g cans chopped tomatoes with garlic

- 200g barbecue sauce (measure by filling half a 400g can if you don't have scales)

- 1 tbsp dried oregano or mixed dried herbs

- x 400g cans pinto beans

- grated cheddar and tortilla chips, to serve (optional)

Method

1. Heat the oil in a large casserole dish with a lid. Add the onion and bacon, and cook over a medium heat for 15 mins, until the onion is really soft and starting to brown, and the bacon is crisp. Push to the side of

the pan, increase the heat and add the chicken pieces. Cook for a few mins until the meat is nicely browned, but don't worry if it's not evenly coloured. Add the paprika, tomatoes, along with half a can (200ml) water, the barbecue sauce, herbs, a pinch of salt and a generous amount of black pepper. Cover with a lid, lower the heat to a gentle simmer and cook for 45 mins, stirring occasionally.

2. Check that the chicken is tender – if not, cover again and cook for 15 mins more. Add the beans and simmer, uncovered, for 20 mins until the sauce is thickened. Serve in bowls topped with grated cheddar and tortilla chips, if you like.